I0410673

Understanding ALCOHOLISM...the baffling disease that HIJACKS the human brain!

Understanding ALCOHOLISM...the baffling disease that HIJACKS the human brain!

KURT N.*

* In keeping with AA's tradition of anonymity, the author's pseudo name has been used.

Copyright © 2016 Kurt N.*
All rights reserved.

ISBN-13: 9781537729183
ISBN-10: 1537729187

Understanding ALCOHOLISM

An easy-to-understand, non- technical guide to understanding this baffling disease!

- Genetic factors….
- Why they just can't stop…
- Role of environment…
- Interventions…
- Treatment programs…
- Available medications…
- Health risks of alcoholism…
- Family recovery programs…
- Where to find help…
- Other resources available…
  And much more…

Dedication

This book is dedicated to the hundreds of recovering alcoholics who have shared various portions of their stories with me over the past 30 years; to the Houston Public Library, which maintains an excellent selection of books and other research materials on alcoholism; and to the dedicated counselors at Serenity House and members of the Virginia Association of Alcoholism and Drug Abuse Counselors, who willingly shared their knowledge of the disease with me.

I would also be remiss if I failed to thank my good friend, Don K., without whose help and encouragement this book would not have been written, and such wonderful organizations as The National Council on Alcoholism and Drug Addiction, Join Together, The National Institute on Alcohol Abuse and Alcoholism, and SAMHSH's National Clearing House for Alcoholism and Drug Information for the vast resources they have made available.

Introduction

If you are wondering if you could be an alcoholic, or are a family member or friend of someone who is having a problem with alcohol, don't feel alone. Experts estimate that some 15 to 20 million Americans abuse alcohol and/or are alcoholics, and perhaps 50 million more are directly affected by their drinking. Yet, it is amazing how little most Americans know about alcoholism.

While this book is not designed to be an exhaustive, scientific treatise on the disease, it is based on the knowledge I have acquired during over 30 years as an active member of Alcoholics Anonymous, attendance at thousands of AA and Al-Anon meetings, over three years working at a major east coast treatment center, and my own personal study of alcoholism, spanning well over two decades.

I believe it will provide you with a better understanding of the insidious, genetically-based disease called alcoholism, what it is, its causes, its treatment, and what you, as either an alcoholic or someone whose life is affected by the actions of an alcoholic can and cannot do about it.

ALCOHOLISM

...one of the world's most misunderstood diseases!

*O*f all the diseases afflicting mankind, perhaps none is more misunderstood that alcoholism. For centuries, man has viewed it as a character defect, or as a sin, or as a lack of willpower, if you will.

Perhaps what makes alcoholism so hard to understand is the fact that an estimated 90% of Americans who drink are able to do so without ever having a problem.

And when you add to this the fact that the behavior of alcoholics often adversely affects the lives of others, it is easy to see why many people have a difficult time viewing alcoholism as a disease rather than simply a behavioral (or character) issue.

And yet, scientific study after scientific study (as you will see shortly) show that **genetics** and not willpower or character determine whether or not a person who drinks will become an alcoholic. Or, to put it simply, the bodies of alcoholics and the way they process alcohol are different from those of the general public.

And both the American Medical Association and the federal government agree that alcoholism is indeed a disease.

Unfortunately, however, the prevailing misconceptions concerning alcoholism are probably still keeping millions of alcoholics from admitting they have a problem and seeking the help they need to deal with it.

After all, how many of us want to be viewed as someone who is simply too "weak-willed" to do anything about his or her drinking? Or even worse, as an "unrepentant sinner," who is unwilling to change his or her way of life?

And so, untreated alcoholism continues to tear up millions of American homes and destroy millions of American lives.

Emphasizing the immensity of the problem, the late Reverend Vernon E. Johnson, founder of the Johnson Institute in Minneapolis, Minnesota, estimated that "*10% of the drinkers in America will become alcoholics.*"

Fortunately as more and more scientists begin to study the disease of alcoholism, these views are beginning to change drastically. Yet there is much to be done.

So if you are a friend or a relative of an alcoholic or someone who seems to be having a problem with alcohol, I urge you to learn as much as possible about the disease of alcoholism and speak out against the ignorance and prejudice that is still keeping so many alcoholics—perhaps someone you know or love--from getting the help they need. It's time to bring alcoholism out of the dark ages!

****

"It is better to light a single candle

than to curse the darkness."

ELEANOR ROOSEVELT

****

*It is my prayer that this little book may serve
as one small candle in shedding new light
upon the baffling disease of alcoholism.*

KURT N.*

****

**At one time people with epilepsy were
considered to be demon-possessed
and were shunned by the public.**

HISTORY OF EPILEPSY,
NORTH DAKOTA STATE UNIVERSITY

****

Alcoholism-- A Deadly Disease!

*U*nfortunately like many other diseases, as Reverend Johnson points out in his well-known book, "I'll Quit Tomorrow'" untreated alcoholism is deadly disease—**"100% fatal"**--and will almost inevitably result in the premature death of the alcoholic.

While it is difficult to come up with exact numbers due to the fact that many doctors are reluctant to name alcoholism as the cause of death for fear of lawsuits, the Center for Disease Control estimates the number of deaths underlined directly attributed to alcoholism at approximately 75,000 a year!

Unfortunately, dying of alcoholism is not the peaceful "dozing-off into eternity" death that many alcoholics assume that it will be. It's a slow, painful, and long-suffering death that grieves both the alcoholic and the entire family.

If you are dealing with an alcoholic, I urge you to do everything in your power to find help for that person as quickly as possible. You are truly dealing with a life and death situation.

Some Frequently-Asked Questions

Following are some of the most frequently-asked questions I have encountered over the years discussing alcoholism with those unfamiliar with the disease. I believe they will help you get a better understanding of this insidious disease.

WHAT DETERMINES IF A PERSON IS AN ALCOHOLIC?

Although there are numerous "tests" one can take to determine if he or she is an alcoholic (See the appendix for some of them), alcoholics generally find that once they start drinking, they have little or no control over the amount they drink.

How often have I heard them say, "*I only intended to have one or two, but once I started, I found myself going back for another and then another. And before the evening was over, I was drunk. It seemed as though once I took that first drink I just couldn't leave it alone **even though I knew what it was going to do to me!***"

In the book, "Alcoholics Anonymous," published by Alcoholics Anonymous World Services, Inc., Dr. William D. Silkworth, one of the great pioneers in the treatment of alcoholism, calls this "*the phenomenon of craving,*" an irresistible physical sensation that occurs once an alcoholic has taken that first or second drink....a sensation "*that never occurs in the average temperate drinker.*"

Obviously then, the bodies and brains of alcoholics react differently to alcohol than the bodies and brains of non-alcoholics.

In fact, if you have ever watched a group of non-`alcoholics drinking, you will realize that the way they drink is entirely different from the way alcoholic friends or family members do. Many non-alcoholics will take a small sip from a glass of wine, for example, and then set it down to enjoy a bit of food or to participate in a conversation, while alcoholics will often quickly drink the entire glass and then order more.

IF THEY CAN'T DRINK NORMALLY, WHY DO THEY DRINK AT ALL?

This is a question that has apparently been troubling non-alcoholics for centuries. In fact, it even seemed to bother King Solomon, reputed to have been the wisest man in the world (See Proverbs 23: 29-35), so it's not surprising that most non-alcoholics do not understand it.

The simple fact is that in many cases, the alcoholic simply cannot help it! Often before they realize it, most alcoholics reach the point where their brains have been "warped" to such an extent that they are literally unable to rationally decide whether to drink or not.

As pointed out in the book "Alcoholics Anonymous, *"At a certain point in the drinking of every alcoholic, he passes into a state where the most powerful desire to stop drinking is of absolutely no avail…The point is that most alcoholics have lost the power of choice in drink"*

As anchorwoman Elizabeth Vargas stated recently on 20/20 in an ABC special with Barbara Walters, *"I would die for my children, I would kill for my children, but I could not stop drinking for my children."*

As David Rosenbloom, PhD, director of Join Together, is quoted in the book, "Addiction—Why Can't They Just Stop?", ***"They can't stop because their brains have been changed!"***

I can well remember that after being hospitalized for alcoholism for the second time, I was determined to quit drinking, for I knew that if I had just one drink I would once again not be able to stop and would suffer the embarrassment of being hospitalized for the third time. Yet within a week, I was drunk again and headed back to the hospital once more.

In recent years, neuroscience through the use of brain imaging has given us valuable new insights to use in developing a better understanding of the disease of alcoholism.

In their excellent book "<u>addiction</u>," Drs. Kevin McCauley and Cory Reich, for example, suggest that "<u>Addiction is a combined genetic-and stress-induced defect in the midbrain and prefrontal cortex dopamine/glutamate reward-learning system, resulting in symptoms of decreased functioning, namely: loss of control, craving, and persistent use of the drug/behavior despite negative consequences.</u>"

Most counselors today will agree that it is irrational to expect rational behavior from one who no longer has the mental ability to act rationally. Call it "insanity" if you will. But if you are dealing with a practicing alcoholic*, you are probably dealing with a mentally sick person who is desperately in need of help.

In the beginning, of course, most alcoholics begin drinking for much the same reason that most other people drink. They like the effect produced by alcohol!

As a "mind-altering drug," it produces a number of chemical changes in the brain that generate a "sense of ease and comfort" that nearly all drinkers–whether alcoholics or not– seem to enjoy.

Due to the large amounts of dopamine being released by alcohol into their systems many alcoholics also report that alcohol gives them a feeling of empowerment, of being able to handle situations they could not handle otherwise...by removing fears, inhibitions and insecurities.

Others claim that it frees their imagination and increases their creative abilities. In fact, the head of a major advertising agency I am personally familiar with once told his copywriters, "*If you write better when you drink, then drink!*" And I know of several very successful advertising campaigns that were conceived while the copywriters were "under the influence."

*The term "practicing alcoholic" refers to one who is currently drinking.

In another example of alcohol's unique effect on alcoholics, Paul Harvey once told of a study conducted by a major university that was designed to show the effect alcohol had on the reaction time of drivers. According to Harvey, there were several students whose reaction time actually improved after one or two drinks instead of decreasing as had been expected.

When they sought to find out what made this group different from the norm, they found that every single person in that group came from a family with a history of alcoholism Of course, after a few more drinks, everyone's reaction time deteriorated considerably, but still the study showed that alcohol affected the students from alcoholic families differently than the others.

Because alcohol does affect alcoholics differently, it is not surprising that many people have been extremely successful in spite of (or perhaps because of) the fact that they were alcoholics or at least "heavy drinkers."

These include Winston Churchill, Ernest Hemingway, and Ulysses S. Grant, to name but a few. In fact, when he was told that General Grant was drinking a bottle a day, President Lincoln is reported to have ordered his aide to find out what brand Grant was drinking, so that he could order a barrel for each of his other generals!

Because of the seemingly positive effects of alcohol, many practicing alcoholics do not seem to recognize drinking as being a problem, but rather as "a solution." And over time, unfortunately, they find it to be a virtually indispensable aid in dealing with the problems and frustrations encountered in everyday life.

In fact, so strong is this dependence on alcohol that it is not unusual for an alcoholic to go through a period of "mourning" when forced to give up drinking. As a recovering alcoholic from North Carolina once told me, "I felt as though I had just lost my best friend. I just didn't know how to handle life without it."

Aren't most alcoholics "skid-row" types?

This is another wide-spread misconception that makes it so difficult for many people to admit that, even though they don't like the idea, they or their loved ones have become alcoholics.

The truth is that most alcoholics (perhaps 90% of those I have known personally) are people that few would ever suspect of ever having had a problem with alcohol.

During the years I have been attending A.A. meetings, I have met hundreds of them, including top executives with major banks and leading corporations, dozens of successful attorneys and physicians, CPAs, former airline pilots, retired judges, a former U.S. Congressman, a former governor, two television stars, engineers, college professors, several Catholic and Episcopal priests, several Catholic nuns, three Methodist ministers, and two Baptist preachers, to name but a few.

And who can forget such well-known personalities as Betty Ford, Mamie Eisenhower, and Edgar Allen Poe, one of America's greatest poets.

Confirming my personal findings, a Survey of Membership conducted by Alcoholics Anonymous found that approximately 11% of members were entrepreneurs, 10% held managerial or administrative positions, 10% were professionals or technicians, 8% were skilled craftsmen, and 5% were health professionals.

And I, myself, have had opportunities to attend several "professional conferences for alcoholics" that were attended by dozens of recovering physicians and attorneys.

Unfortunately, however, many of those who are now on "skid row" were also once respected members of their communities until alcohol robbed them of their careers and self-respect.

Is alcoholism hereditary?

Unfortunately, it certainly appears to be. Over the years, I have found that almost invariably alcoholics come from families that had problems with alcohol.

Researchers who have studied this field have also found that there is substantial evidence that shows beyond any reasonable doubt that one's potential of becoming an alcoholic is indeed genetic.

Psychiatrist and researcher, Dr. Donald Goodwin, for example, found that children of alcoholics–even though raised by non-alcoholic adoptive or foster parents--have *a four-times higher rate of alcoholism* than children of non-alcoholics, <u>in spite of the fact that they had no contact with the alcoholic parent(s) after the first few weeks of life!</u>

He also found that children of non-alcoholic parents– even though raised by alcoholic adoptive or foster parents–had relatively low rates of alcoholism.

Extensive research by others, including Charles Lieber, chief of the research program on liver disease and nutrition at the Bronx VA Hospital; and psychiatrist and researcher Marc Schuckit, of the University of California in San Diego, has also shown that physiology (not character or willpower) is the determining factor in whether or not a person will become an alcoholic.

And a report released in February, 2006 by The National Council on Alcoholism and Drug Dependence states that: "*recent neurobiological, genetic, pharmacological and brain imaging research*" also indicates that alcoholism is indeed a <u>genetically predisposed disease.</u> Unfortunately, however, trying to isolate and identify the alcoholic gene (or genes) has proven to be extremely difficult. In fact, a report recently released by the National Institute on Alcohol Abuse and Alcoholism classifies alcoholism as <u>a complex, multi-genetic disease</u> "*influenced by <u>many genes</u> located in different areas of a person's DNA.*"

Further intensifying the genetic predisposition to alcoholism is the fact that children from alcoholic homes almost invariably marry one another. Almost without exception, every married alcoholic I know is married either to another alcoholic, or, if not to an alcoholic, to someone from an alcoholic home.

It is interesting to note that one's ethnic background also seems to be an indicator of the probability of one becoming an alcoholic, again confirming the genetic link.

Of the thousands of alcoholics I have known over the years, I am aware of only four that came from ethnically-pure Jewish families, three or four with Italian backgrounds, and three who were Orientals. Yet I have known hundreds whose ancestors came from northern Europe, as well as hundreds of Blacks and Hispanics.

Join Together, a national clearing house for information on alcoholism, also recently reported a study that found that the alcoholism rate among Native Americans is <u>six</u> <u>times</u> the national average!

In his excellent book, "<u>The Emergent Comprehensive Concept of Alcoholism</u>," researcher and author James R. Milam discusses the correlation between the length of time an ethnic group has been exposed to alcohol and the rate of alcoholism in that group.

As Milam points out, Italians and Jews have had alcohol available for well over 7,000 years as compared to less than 2,000 years for most Northern Europeans, while American Indians were first exposed to alcohol only a few centuries ago. Researchers theorize that over the centuries, natural selection has continuously reduced the percentage of those who are genetically predisposed to alcoholism within the various ethnic groups.

DOES THIS MEAN THAT CHILDREN OF ALCOHOLICS ARE DESTINED TO BECOME ALCOHOLICS?

Of course not! Even though they may be genetically predisposed toward alcoholism, it does not necessarily mean that they are destined to become alcoholics. Whether or not they will ever develop "*the phenomenon of craving*" that defines an alcoholic depends upon of the level of their **genetic predisposition** and the amount they need to drink before becoming physically addicted.

Some are so "pre-programmed" physiologically that they will become alcoholics almost from the time they pick up the first drink. Other will be able to drink more or less normally for years before the phenomenon of craving that defines an alcoholic sets in.

However, since children of alcoholics are frequently allowed to sample alcohol at an early age, many will also begin drinking while in their teens (or even earlier), thus increasing the probability that they, too, will become both physically and psychologically addicted.

Stressing the correlation between alcoholism and environment, research recently released by the Substance Abuse and Mental Health Services Administration stated that 88% of the people in treatment first got drunk before their 21st birthday, with 12% first getting drunk before the age of 12, and 25% admitting getting drunk for the first time before the age of 14.

Unfortunately in many cultures, including the one in which I was raised, parents often allow small children to have a sip or two (or more) out of their glasses, thus introducing them to alcohol before reaching the age of 2 or 3 without realizing the danger of doing so.

The important role that environment can play was also pointed out in a study published in the December, 2003 issue of the <u>Archives of General Psychiatry</u> which found that, *"family environment effects do make a difference in accounting for offspring outcomes, in particular, that a low-risk environment (i.e. the absence of parental alcoholism) can moderate the impact of high genetic risk regarding offspring for the development of alcohol-use disorders."*

Or, as the saying goes, "While it's genetics that load the gun, it's usually the environment that pulls the trigger!"

As science has not yet been able to determine the extent of one's genetic predisposition, the safest course for those with alcoholism anywhere in their family of origin is not to drink at all, and certainly not to allow children to drink at any age.

NOTE: It is a common misconception that when preparing dishes which include wine or other alcoholic beverages as part of the recipe that the alcohol will "be cooked out." However, according to a recent article by the famous chef and chemist, Joe LaVilla (who in addition to graduating from the Culinary Institute of America also holds a PhD in organic chemistry from the University of Rochester), **up to 60% of the alcohol can remain in a dish even after cooking!** The safest bet is to substitute grape juice or other non-alcoholic ingredients.

NEITHER OF MY PARENTS WERE ALCOHOLICS, SO I COULDN'T POSSIBLY BE ONE. RIGHT?

How I wish that were true! However, as the book, "Alcoholics Anonymous," points out, alcoholism is "a cunning and baffling disease," and so it is not unusual for it to skip one or more generations. Take my own case for example:

To the best of my knowledge, neither my mother nor my father ever had a problem with alcohol. In fact, except for holidays and wedding receptions, I cannot remember ever seeing my mother take a drink. And although my father would have a few beers from time to time, I never once saw him drunk. Yet both my brother and I carried the alcoholism gene(s) and eventually became alcoholics. The simple fact is that although my parents carried the alcoholism gene(s), they never drank enough to "kick off" the disease of alcoholism.

However I do remember that my mother's father loved to drink In fact to assure a constant supply, he planted his own vineyard and produced huge vats of wine each year, storing it in 50-gallon barrels in the cellar. He also kept a supply of whiskey hidden throughout the basement. (And his brother died of cirrhosis of the liver in Austria...also not a good sign!)

I can also remember going to the bar with my grandfather as a child and watching him drink "boilermakers," while I sipped on coke and played the pinball machines. And although no one dared mention the word, "alcoholic" in our family because of its negative connotations at the time, my mother would not allow one of my father's brothers to come to our house because of his "excessive drinking."

So even if neither of your parents were alcoholics—or even "heavy drinkers"—you could still very well carry the alcoholism gene (or genes).

A far better question to ask yourself is: "Is there evidence of alcoholism <u>anywhere</u> in my family of origin?" If so, even though you don't like the idea, you could be (or become) an alcoholic. If so, "welcome to the club!" Trust me; it's not the end of the world! There is help.

Are all heavy drinkers alcoholics?

No. And this has led to a great deal of confusion and frustration among family members and friends of alcoholics.

Nearly everyone knows or has heard of "a heavy drinker" who one day decided that alcohol was causing too many problems in his or her life and so simply stopped drinking or limited the amount consumed to a point where it did not produce any adverse effects.

This makes it difficult for people to understand why the alcoholic in their life can't do the same thing.

To further compound the confusion, many who are destined to become alcoholics will be able to properly control their drinking for years before they become physically and mentally addicted to alcohol.

Why does this difference exist?

The determining factor seems to be the body's ability to process alcohol without producing certain chemical compounds that alter brain chemistry and function enough to produce the <u>irresistible</u> craving mentioned earlier. And this seems to be directly related to the varying quantities of certain enzymes each person's body produces.

A report issued in July, 2003, by the National Institute on Alcohol Abuse and Alcoholism stated in part: "*One well character-ized relationship between genes and alcoholism is the result of varia-tions in the <u>liver enzymes </u>that metabolize (breakdown) alcohol....The genes for these <u>enzymes</u> and the alleles, or gene variants that alter alcohol metabolism have been identified.*"

As with most substances produced by the human body, the quantity of these enzymes can vary considerably from person to person, and usually declines with age.

Individuals whose bodies produce relatively few of the enzymes required to effectively (and safely) process alcohol will often become physically and mentally addicted shortly after they start drinking.

Others will be able to drink safely for years until their bodies stop producing sufficient quantities and then they, too, will find themselves craving alcohol after taking the first or second drink.

Then there will also be those whose bodies produce so many of these enzymes that they will never experience that irresistible "phenomenon of craving" that defines an alcoholic no matter how much they drink. And these seem to be the "heavy drinkers" who can stop at will.

I'VE BEEN ARRESTED FOR DRUNKEN DRIVING. DOES THAT MEAN I AM AN ALCOHOLIC?

Not necessarily. Yet it is a good indication that you may have a problem with alcohol. It has been my experience that most men and women who are arrested for driving under the influence have been doing so for quite some time before being arrested.

The important question is: Are you truly able to effectively control your drinking, limiting yourself to one or two when necessary? (I urge you to be honest.) If you can, you may well just be "a heavy drinker," and hopefully you have learned your lesson and won't get behind the wheel of a car again in the same condition again.

Of course, if you believe that you <u>are</u> able to control your drinking, you have to ask yourself <u>why</u> you drank so much that you deliberately put yourself and others in danger. And this is a question that only you can answer.

If you have to admit that you have driven while intoxicated more than once--or this is the second or third time you have been arrested--I urge you to get help before you kill or seriously injure yourself or another person.

I have a friend in AA who failed to heed this warning and wound up killing his young son in a wreck he caused while driving drunk. Needless to say, neither he nor his wife has ever gotten over it. I urge you not to take the risk. If you can't afford a treatment center, call AA or one of the other 12-step programs mentioned in the back under "Other Resources". These programs are free and they could save your life or the life of someone you care about.

CAN ALCOHOLISM BE CURED?

To the best of my knowledge, nothing has been found so far that can turn an alcoholic into a normal drinker. It seems that once a person has experienced the so-called "phenomenon of craving," it becomes impossible for him or her to ever drink normally again. The only solution appears to be complete abstinence.

By this time, however, most alcoholics have also become so psychologically addicted to alcohol that they find it almost impossible to leave it alone without outside help.

CAN ALCOHOLISM BE EFFECTIVELY TREATED?

Yes! Fortunately the disease of alcoholism can usually be arrested if the alcoholic truly has a desire to stop drinking.

Perhaps the best-known treatment program for alcoholics is *Alcoholics Anonymous*, which to date has helped millions of alcoholics learn how to live sober, happy, and productive lives.

Although most treatment centers I am familiar with offer significant (and often vital) additional services and counseling, nearly all base their programs around the 12 steps of the *Alcoholics Anonymous* program.

Additional information on the AA program and on other programs dealing with alcoholism can be obtained by contacting the appropriate resources listed at the back of this book.

How successful are treatment programs?

If by "successful," you mean that alcoholics who enter treatment and/or join A.A. or other programs remain sober for the rest of their lives, then the answer would have to be that most programs have a very low rate of success...perhaps as low as 10% to 15%.

However, Mark Willenbring, MD,, of the National Institute on Alcohol Abuse and Alcoholism, reports that the recovery rate of alcoholics who receive treatment is very encouraging, with some two-thirds of them recovering over time.

Most all alcoholics I have known personally (perhaps the vast majority) have also gone back to drinking one or more times before achieving any substantial length of sobriety. However, many of them have now been sober for many years and may well stay sober for the rest of their lives. In fact I know of several who have been sober for 30, 40, even 50 years.

The book <u>Alcoholics Anonymous,</u> however, (probably the best-known book in the world on alcoholism) maintains that those who "thoroughly follow" the AA program will "almost invariably get well". And I also believe this to be true.

Unfortunately, however, not all alcoholics are willing to "thoroughly follow" the AA program, which calls for taking actions that are directly contrary to our basic human nature.

These include admitting that they are absolutely powerless over alcohol, making a searching and fearless moral inventory of their lives, making a list of all persons they have harmed, making amends to them wherever possible, and helping other alcoholics without any thought of reward.

And so many will try to stay sober solely on the support and fellowship they find at AA meetings. Surprisingly, some of them will be able to stay sober in this manner for years. But I have found that most will go back to drinking within a few months.

I have talked to dozens of them over the years...men and women who claimed that they "had tried the AA program" and that "*it just hadn't worked*" for them.

Yet nearly all of them later admitted that they hadn't actually taken the actions suggested by the program but had only been going to meetings.

As an old AA friend recently put it: "*Just going to meetings and then complaining the program didn't work for you is like going into a restaurant and refusing to order or to eat any of the food being offered and then complaining that the restaurant just didn't fill you up.*"

Another problem many have is the tendency of the human mind to enhance the memories of pleasant experiences and diminish the memories of unpleasant ones. Thus after a period of sobriety, they remember the pleasurable experiences they had while drinking and forget or minimize the misery that alcohol caused them and others.

Then, too, many alcoholics do not seem to realize the seriousness of the disease, and treat it as cavalierly as if it were just a bad cold. Yet alcoholism, as I have stated before, is <u>a deadly</u> <u>disease</u>. I know because I have attended the funerals of several alcoholics, including family members, who literally drank themselves to death.

IF ALCOHOLISM IS A DISEASE, WOULDN'T DOCTORS BE THE IDEAL ONES TO TREAT IT?

In an ideal world, yes. Unfortunately we have found that few doctors have any real understanding of the disease and few have received sufficient training to be of any real value.

The son-in-law of an old AA friend in Houston, for example, once told him that in eight years of medical school, he had spent only one afternoon studying the disease of alcoholism.

And so, whenever he encountered a patient who seemed to have a problem with alcohol, his standard procedure was to call his father-in-law and ask him how to handle it.

Then, too, there is the problem of time. Alcoholism is a complex disease involving not only the body but the mind of the alcoholic as well. And with their busy schedules, probably few doctors have the time required to properly treat and counsel alcoholics.

However, doctors can play an important role by explaining the tremendous toll that alcohol is having on the human body and the fatal nature of the disease and encouraging alcoholics to seek treatment. I personally know of several AA members who sought treatment at the urging of their physicians.

AREN'T THERE ANY MEDICATIONS THAT CAN HELP TREAT ALCOHOLISM?

Although science has not yet been able to develop one that can cure or permanently arrest the disease, there are several medications that have proven to be very useful in the treatment of alcoholism.

Medications such as **Librium** and **Valium** are often used during the first few days after alcoholics stop drinking to help them safely withdraw from alcohol. However they are also highly addictive, and so they are normally not used over an extended period of time.

Other medications include **Naltrexone,** which can help reduce the craving for alcohol, **Antabuse**, which makes most people feel sick if they drink, and **Acamprosate**, which is believed to help modulate and normalize alcohol-related changes in brain activity, thereby reducing symptoms of protracted withdrawal, such as disturbances in sleep patterns and moods that may trigger a relapse into drinking.

<u>Naltrexone</u> is also now available in extended-release injectable form, which helps solve the problem of patient noncompliance.

A newcomer to the pharmacological arsenal available to help in the treatment of alcoholism is a drug called **gabapentin**, which is approved by the FDA for treating epilepsy and neuropathic pain.

A recent 12-week study, showed that **gabapentin** not only decreased the number of days participants receiving the drug drank heavily, but also at least tripled the percentage of people who were able to stop drinking altogether, as compared to those receiving a placebo.

As nearly all medications can have undesirable (and often dangerous) side effects, they should only be used on the advice of physicians.

Another problem with medications seems to be that they do little, if anything, to relieve the alcoholic's psychological addiction to alcohol. I have had several alcoholics tell me over the years that when they wanted to once again experience the temporary "feeling of ease and comfort" that alcohol always seemed to provide, they simply stopped taking their medications and went back to drinking.

As my professional friends tell me, medications alone are not "a magic bullet," but can be "helpful" when used in conjunction with a strong counseling program.

WHAT ARE THE HEALTH RISKS OF ALCOHOLISM?

Although "having a few drinks per day" does appear to have certain health benefits, the effects of excessive drinking can be devastating, often leading to insanity and/or premature death.

The U.S. Center for Disease Control and Prevention reports that not only does alcohol kill an estimated 75,000 Americans each year, but it cuts their lives short by an average of 30 years!

And if one needs further evidence of the fatal nature of untreated alcoholism, the June 27, 2009 issue of <u>The Lancet</u> reports that a study by the Russian Cancer Research Center found that *"more than half of the deaths of Russians ages 15 to 54 were attributable to alcohol consumption during the 10-year period following the collapse of the Soviet Union in late 1991."*

Following are some of the effects alcohol can have on major organs of the body as reported by various medical studies…

The Brain: Although most people realize that alcohol destroys brain cells, few are aware of the tremendous toll it can have on the brain. In addition to adversely affecting memory and concentration, long-term alcohol consumption can also lead to a condition known as "alcoholic insanity" or "wet brain," a condition in which so many brain cells have been destroyed that the alcoholic loses the ability to perform even such routine tasks as feeding him-or-herself or using the toilet. And once alcoholics reach that stage, there appears to be no way of reviving these skills.

To illustrate the effects of alcohol on the human brain, researchers at Wellesley College used MRI scans to measure the brain size of 1800 drinkers and non-drinkers. They reported that people who consumed 14 or more alcoholic drinks <u>per week</u> had brains that were an average of 1.6% smaller than those of nondrinkers.

When you consider that most alcoholics drink far in excess of that amount (many will drink 14 to 28 or more drinks <u>per day</u>), you can easily imagine the effect of chronic alcoholism on the human brain.

The Liver: As the liver is primarily responsible for the proper processing of alcohol, it is also unfortunately the organ most seriously affected by it. In addition to cirrhosis of the liver (irreversible scarring, lesions, and the destruction of liver cells), alcoholism can also cause alcoholic hepatitis, and a condition known as edema (the building up of fluid in the extremities), and yellow jaundice. These conditions often lead to complete liver failure, which can produce comas and death.

The Heart: Although moderate alcohol consumption has been shown to be beneficial to the heart, excessive drinking can also damage the heart muscle (cardiomyopathy) reducing the heart's ability to properly pump blood, leading to abnormal heart function. It is also believed to be a major cause of heart failure, increased blood pressure, and stroke.

In addition to affecting these and other key organs, alcohol has also been shown to be a major factor in the development of many other serious health problems that are plaguing millions of Americans today. These include:

Breast Cancer: Not surprisingly, considering its effect on other parts of the body, alcohol has also been shown to be a major contributing factor in the development of breast cancer.

An article appearing in the March 15, 2007 issue of the American Journal of Epidemiology, reports that after studying data on some 39,000 women, Harvard researchers found that women who drink 30 grams (about 1 oz.) or more of alcohol per day have a 43% greater chance of developing breast cancer than non-drinkers!

Sexual Dysfunction (including impotence): According to reports published by the National Institute on Alcohol Abuse and Alcoholism, alcohol abuse has also been associated with sexual dysfunction and a loss of libido in both men and women. In addition, alcohol abuse in men has been shown to cause impaired testosterone production and shrinkage of the testes, leading to impotence, infertility, and reduced male sexual characteristics.

The National Institute for Alcohol Abuse and Alcoholism also reports that alcohol can affect female reproductive organs. According to NIAAA, adolescent girls who consume even moderate amounts of alcohol may experience disrupted growth and puberty, while excessive alcohol use by adult women can cause infertility, increase risk of spontaneous abortion, and impaired fetal growth and development.

In addition, even moderate alcohol use during pregnancy has also been found to be major cause of behavior problems in children. According to a report published on December 3, 2008 by <u>Reuters Health</u>, researchers found that *"women who consume even one drink weekly while pregnant are more likely to have children with behavior problems than women who abstain."* The study found that 44% of the mothers diagnosed with alcoholism who drank during pregnancy had children with conduct disorders, <u>more than twice the rate</u> of alcoholic mothers who abstained while pregnant.

Osteoporosis: Excessive alcohol consumption has also been found to be a major factor in the development of osteoporosis, often leading to fragile bones, fractured hips, and loss of height in both men and women. In a recent report, H. Wayne Sampson, PhD, professor of human anatomy and medical neurobiology and nutrition at Texas A&M University, states that: *"Both human and animal studies clearly indicate that chronic heavy drinking, particularly during adolescent and young adult years, can dramatically compromise bone quality and may increase osteoporosis risk."*

Alzheimer's: Considering the fact that excessive drinking frequently produces "blackouts" (a period of time of which the drinker has absolutely no recollections of his actions or activities), it is not surprising that it is also credited with the early onset of Alzheimer's disease.

According to an article appearing recently in "<u>Health Day News</u>", a recent study of people 60-years old and older who were diagnosed with possible or probable Alzheimer's found that the onset of the disease for those drinking more than two drinks a day was an average of 4.8 years earlier than for more "moderate" or non-drinkers.

Severe Memory Impairment: Even if one is fortunate enough not to suffer from Alzheimer's, chances are good that alcoholics will still face the real possibility of having to deal with severe memory impairment.

According to an article appearing in the June 9th, 2014 issue of Geriatric Medicine, a study which covered over 6,000 middle-aged adults for up to 19 years found that those with "alcohol use disorders" had more than doubled their chances of suffering from "severe memory impairment" later in life.

Skin Cancer (including melanoma): According to a recent study reported in the British Journal of Dermatology, alcohol consumption can also play a major role in the development of skin cancer, including the development of melanoma, the deadliest form of skin cancer.

In examining 16 studies involving thousands of participants, researchers found that having at least one alcoholic drink daily increases the risk of skin cancer by 20%, and people who drank the equivalent of a few strong beers daily were 55% more likely to develop melanoma, as compared to people who didn't drink or who drank only occasionally..

Other Effects: As if those already mentioned were not enough, The Journal for the Society for the Study of Addiction recently published a report that stated that, *"…the epidemiological evidence can support the judgement that alcohol causes cancer of the oropharynx, larynx, esophagus, liver, colon, rectum and breast."*

Excessive alcohol consumption has also been found to affect the lungs, the intestines, the pancreas, the stomach, joints (arthritis), muscles (atrophy), and estrogen metabolism.

Researchers also consider it to be a major factor in causing such health problems as ulcers, kidney failure, lung collapse, acid reflux, and nerve damage (peripheral neuropathy).

CAN YOU CAUSE SOMEONE TO BECOME AN ALCOHOLIC?

The answer is no! Not unless you are able to change their genetic makeup, which obviously you are not. I would like to emphasis once again that alcoholism is a metabolic, hereditary, generic **disease**!

Yet this question is often asked by spouses, parents, and other relatives and friends of alcoholics. And no wonder. For before going into recovery, it is not unusual for alcoholics to blame others for their drinking. And sadly most of them sincerely believe what they are saying, so clever is the human mind in justifying irrational behavior.

How often have I heard them say: *"If it weren't for my wife (or my boss, or my job, etc.), I wouldn't have to drink like this!"* And I know that at the time, they sincerely believed what they were saying. Yet, after a period of sobriety, most were willing to admit that they were wrong. In fact, many of them still had the same wife and the same job and the same boss several years later and were leading happy, successful, sober lives.

The simple fact is that no one can cause an alcoholic to drink without either pouring it down his or her throat or holding a gun to his or her head.

CAN YOU CONTROL AN ALCOHOLIC'S DRINKING?

Unfortunately, in most cases, you cannot. Tactics, such as pouring out or watering down liquor, seldom, if ever, work. Nor do frothy emotional appeals. Once a person has crossed the line into alcoholism, he or she will normally go to any length to obtain and guard his or her supply, including lying, hiding bottles, stealing, pawning jewelry or other personal items, taking out loans, or whatever else it might take.

In fact the lengths to which alcoholics will go to in order to do so will often amaze non-alcoholics.

An alcoholic I knew in Texas, for example, told me that he once drained the windshield washer fluid out of his car, filled the container with vodka and then connected a rubber tube and ran it under the dashboard, so that whenever he wanted a drink, he could simply place the tube in his mouth and turn on the windshield washer.

How can you make an alcoholic seek help?

Before you can get an alcoholic to seek or accept help, he or she must <u>want</u> help. Yet, because most alcoholics do not see alcohol as being their problem, but rather as their solution to dealing with the frustrations encountered in everyday life, getting them to want help can be extremely difficult.

In fact, as Dr. Silkworth explains it, "*The sensation* (produced by alcohol) *is so elusive that while they admit it is injurious, they cannot after a time differentiate the true from the false. <u>To them their alcoholic life seems the only normal one</u>.*"

Having been associated with alcoholics for over 30 years, I have only seen two factors that sometimes seem to be effective in bringing an alcoholic to the point of actually wanting help:

#1. Love: Sometimes if alcoholics are truly aware of the terrible toll that their drinking is having on the family (particularly on the children), they will be willing to agree to seek help. I know of one alcoholic, for example, who was "*brought to tears*" and finally decided to seek treatment after he overheard his young daughter on the telephone telling a friend that "*her daddy probably wouldn't be there to see her in the play because he probably would be at home drunk again.*"

I knew another AA member who agreed to seek help only after he came home one day to find his wife had set his clothes outside the door and had changed the locks on their house.

Unfortunately, however I also know of several who have walked off from their families, because their physical and psychological addiction to alcohol was so strong that they were absolutely unable to stop regardless of the cost.

(Remember, if you will, that over time, excessive drinking literally hijacks the brain, and many of these simply no longer had the ability to stop drinking, no matter how much they wanted to.

They had in fact lost the power of choice.)

#2. Pain (or the fear of pain): There is an old saying in Alcoholics Anonymous that no alcoholic ever develops a desire to stop drinking until the price he or she is paying to do so becomes too high. For some this may be the loss of a job (or the threat thereof) or deteriorating health. For others it may be emotional pain or the loss of self-respect. For others it may take months or even years of living on the street and/or repeatedly spending time in jails or prisons.

Unfortunately well-meaning family members and friends will often try to protect alcoholics from the consequences of their drinking by lying to employers and friends, providing money, food, and shelter, bailing them out of jail, providing them with legal assistance, etc. And by doing so, they may enable them to continue drinking, often to the point of no return...and death!

Isn't there anything one can do?

Fortunately, yes! In the 1960's the Reverend Vernon Johnson challenged the idea of the prevailing theory that it was impossible to help alcoholics until they had reached their so called "bottom" (a state of "surrender" that usually occurred only after they had lost their families, jobs, finances, or other means of support).

To encourage alcoholics to seek help before reaching this stage, he developed a method of "intervention" that was designed to penetrate their wall of denial and help them become willing to accept professional help.

In an intervention (preferably headed by a trained professional), family members, and often friends and employers gather together and confront the alcoholic about his or her drinking and the effect it is having on everyone involved ...including the alcoholic!

In explaining how an intervention is designed to work, Johnson emphasized the importance of empathetic listening and described it as a form of counseling that is *"more compassionate than aggressive."*

As Johnson explains, "*The goal of the intervention is to have the alcoholic see and accept enough reality so that, however grudgingly, he can in turn accept his need for help. It is not punishment. It is not an opportunity for others to clobber him or her verbally. It is an attack on the victim's wall of defenses, not upon the victim as a person.*"

The "Johnson Model" however, is only one of several models of interventions available to trained interventionists.

Another popular model is the "Family Systemic Invitational Model," which involves the entire family in the recovery process. It is based on the premise that Alcoholism is "a family disease," and it is designed to help all members of the family recover from the effects of alcoholism.

Other types of interventions that have proven popular in recent years include Motivational Enhancement Therapy and Cognitive Behavioral Therapy. Additional information on various intervention programs can be found at www.jointogether.org.

How successful are interventions?

Properly orchestrated, rehearsed, and executed, interventions have generally proven to be highly effective in getting alcoholics to agree to seek and accept help. In fact, success rates of over 90% in getting alcoholics into treatment programs have been reported.

However, whether or not alcoholics who enter treatment via intervention are more successful–or even as successful-- in achieving long-term sobriety has often been debated.

Some professionals I have known feel that patients entering treatment as a result of interventions harbor a great deal of anger and resentment that must be dealt with before the patient is willing to accept help.

Interventionists, however, maintain that if an intervention is done properly, most patients enter treatment programs willingly.

I have personally heard several sober members of the AA program say that an intervention saved their lives. And I also know of several alcoholics who literally drank themselves to death because members of their families failed to do anything!

In his best-selling book, "Intervention," Reverend Johnson maintains that an intervention that is properly done "*always has some effect, and that effect is invariably positive. There is no way it can ever make things worse. At the very least it offers a chance for recovery where before none existed.*"

How do you find an interventionist?

Local treatment centers often have a trained interventionist on staff or can put you in touch with one in your area.

In addition, you may wish to contact the Association of Intervention Specialists for a list of its members in your area. (See "Other Resources" at the back of this book for contact information.)

Since interventions can often "backfire" if handled incorrectly, I would strongly recommend seeking professional help if considering an intervention.

I also highly recommend reading a copy of Reverend Johnson's excellent book, "Intervention," before making your decision. Since you are truly dealing with a life and death matter, interventions are not something to jump into without a great deal of preparation.

ANY OTHER SUGGESTIONS?

YES! If you are a spouse, another family member or friend of someone who has a problem with alcohol, I would strongly recommend actively participating in a family support program.

Two that I am personally familiar with are **Al-Anon** and **Alateen**, both of which are designed to help family members (and friends) cope with the problems so often encountered when living with and/or dealing with alcoholics.

Often recommended by physicians, psychiatrists, and ministers, both programs offer support and information that can prove immensely helpful not only to those participating, but often to the alcoholic as well.

As Joan K. Jackson, Ph.D. explains in the book, "Al-Anon Faces Alcoholism:"

"It is no longer possible to consider alcoholism as a disease affecting only the alcoholic....The relationship between the alcoholic and the family is not a one-way relationship....It is now believed that the most successful treatment of alcoholism involves helping both the alcoholic and those members of the family who are directly involved in the alcoholic's behavior."

Dr. Randolph P. Holmes of Bright Medical Associates, Whittier, Colorado, another ardent supporter of the Al-Anon and Alateen programs, has also found these programs to be a tremendous aid to his patients.

According to Dr. Holmes, *"People who have tried Al-Anon come back to the office more relaxed. It's as if a big burden has been lifted from their chest. They are taking better care of themselves and seem to be enjoying life more, even if the alcoholic goes back to drinking. All in all, I've found few treatments that have given me more satisfaction than a recommendation to attend Al-Anon."*

Having been an active member of Al-Anon myself for several years, I can personally recommend both of these programs to you. In addition to greatly enhancing the quality of the non-alcoholics' lives, I have noticed that when all members of the family are involved in similar programs, most marriages seem to be much stronger and happier.

Information on both of these groups can be found by calling 1-888-4AL-ANON (1-888-425-2666), or by visiting their website www.al-anon.alateen.org.

Appendix

Tests for Alcoholism

Although there are literally dozens of tests one can take to determine whether or not one may be an alcoholic, following are four that I believe are the simplest and most reliable:

Test One

Suggested by the National Institute on Alcohol Abuse and Alcoholism

Q. Have you ever felt you should cut down on your drinking?

Q. Have people annoyed you by criticizing your drinking?

Q. Have you ever felt bad or guilty about your drinking?

Q. Have you ever had a drink first thing in the morning to steady your nerves or to get rid of a hangover?

One "yes" answer suggests a possible alcohol problem.
More than one "yes" answer means it is highly likely
that a problem exists.

Test Two

A popular test developed years ago in the Chicago area, based on information found in "12 Steps and 12 Traditions," a basic text of the AA program.

To determine whether or not you have passed the point of "no return," see if you are still able to control your drinking. The procedure is to drink just two ounces of alcohol each evening, and then not touch a drop until the next evening, at which time you will drink only two ounces again. Try to keep this up for at least a week.

If you find yourself unable to control your drinking in this manner, you are probably an alcoholic.

Test Three
A simple 4-question test developed by SAMHSA's
National Clearing House for Alcohol and Drug Information

Q. Do you ever experience "the sensation of craving" ...a strong, irresistible compulsion to have another drink?

Q. Have you ever lost the ability to control your drinking, drinking far more than you intended to?

Q. Have you ever experienced withdrawal symptoms, such as nausea, sweating, shakiness, and anxiety when the use of alcohol was stopped after a period of heavy drinking?

Q. Do you find that you need to keep drinking greater amounts of alcohol in order to "get high"?

If you answered "yes" **to any of these questions**, chances are good that you may well have a problem with alcohol.

Test Four
*Based on the Alcohol Use Disorders Identification Test
Developed for the World Health Organization, 1992*

1. **How often do you have a drink containing alcohol?**
    (a) Never   (b) Monthly or less   (c) 2-4 times a month
    (d) 2-3 times a week   (e) 4 or more times a week
2. **How many drinks containing alcohol do you have on a typical day when drinking?**
    (a) 1 or 2   (b) 3 or 4   (c) 5 or 6   (d) 7 to 9
    (e) 10 or more
3. **How often do you have 6 or more drinks on one occasion?**
    (a) Never   (b) Less than monthly   (c) Monthly
    (d) Weekly   (e) Daily or Almost Daily
4. **How often during the past year have you found that you were not able to stop drinking once you had started?**
    (a) Never   (b) Less than monthly   (c) Monthly
    (d) Weekly   (e) Daily or Almost Daily
5. **How often during the past year have you failed to do what normally was expected of you because of your drinking?**
    (a) Never   (b) Less than monthly   (c) Monthly
    (d) Weekly   (e) Daily or Almost Daily
6. **How often during the past year have you needed a drink in the morning to get yourself going after a heavy drinking session?**
    (a) Never   (b) Less than monthly   (c) Monthly
    (d) Weekly   (e) Daily or Almost Daily

7. **How often during the last year have you had a feeling of guilt or remorse after drinking?**
   (a) Never   (b) Less than monthly   (c) Monthly
   (d) Weekly   (e) Daily or Almost Daily

8. **How often during the last year have you been unable to remember what happened the night before because of your drinking?**
   (a) Never   (b) Less than monthly   (c) Monthly
   (d) Weekly   (e(Daily or Almost Daily

9. **Have you or someone else been injured because of your drinking?**
   (a) No   (c) Yes, but not in the last year
   (e) Yes, during the last year

10. **Has anyone been concerned about your drinking and/or suggested that you cut down?**
    (a) No   (c) Yes, but not in the last year
    (e) Yes, during the last year

SCORING

Number of (a)'s..............._____ x 0 points = _____

Number of (b)'s..............._____ x 1 point = _____

Number of (c)'s..............._____ x 2 points = _____

Number of (d)'s..............._____ x 3 points = _____

Number of (e)'s..............._____ x 4 points = _____

Your Score: _____

According to the World Health Organization, a score of 8 or more indicates "a strong likelihood of hazardous or harmful alcohol consumption".

Other Resources

Alcoholics Anonymous General Service Office
Box 459, Grand Central Station
New York, N.Y. 10163
Tel: (212) 870-3400
www.aa.org

Al-Anon Family Group Headquarters, Inc.
1600 Corporate Landing Parkway
Virginia Beach, VA 23454-5617
Tel: (888) 425-2666)
www.al-anon.alateen.org

Alcoholics Victorious
Tel: (816) 561-0567
www.alcoholicsvictorious.org

Celebrate Recovery
Tel: (800) 723-3532
www.celebraterecovery.com

Smart Recovery
7537 Mentor Avenue, Suite 306
Mentor, OH 44060
Tel: (866) 951-5357
www.smartrecovery.org

Alcoholics for Chris
1316 N. Campbell Road

Royal Oak, MI 48067
www.alcoholicsforchrist.com

Join Together
"A national clearing house for information regarding recent tests
and developments in the field of alcoholism treatment.
www.jointogether.org

National Institute on Alcohol Abuse and Alcoholism
5635 Fishers Lane, MSC 9304
Bethesda, MD 20892-9304
www.niaaa.nih.gov

The National Council on Alcoholism
And Drug Addiction
244 East 58th Street. 4th Floor
New York, NY 10022
Tel: (212) 269-7797
www.ncadd.org

SAMHSH's National Clearing House
For Alcohol and Drug Information
P.O. Box 2345
Rockville, MD 20847-2345

Association of Intervention Specialists
313 West Liberty Street, Ste. 129
Lancaster, PA 17603 Tel.: (717) 392-8488
www.associationofinterventionspecialists.org

Recommended Reading

"Alcoholics Anonymous"
A.A. World Services

"12 Steps and 12 Traditions"
A.A. World Services

"Under the Influence"
By Dr. James R. Milam
and Katherine Ketcham

"Tough Love"
By Phyllis and David York
and Ted Wachtel

"The Enabler"
By Angelyn Miller, MA

"Intervention"
By Vernon E. Johnson, D.D.

"Al-Anon Faces Alcoholism"
Al-Anon Family Groups
Virginia Beach, VA

"Paths to Recovery"
Al-Anon Family Groups

**"How Al-Anon Works
for families and friends of Alcoholics"**
Al-Anon Family Groups

"addiction"
By Dr. Kevin McCauley and Dr. Cory Reich

"Addiction—Why Can't They Just Stop?"
From Rodale Inc.

"I'll Quit Tomorrow"
By Vernon E. Johnson, D.D.

Understanding ALCOHOLISM!
...the baffling disease that hijacks the human brain!

Presenting answers to questions such as these:

- What is alcoholism?
- Why does he drink so much?
- Why does she drink at all?
- How can I control his drinking?
- Can alcoholism be cured?
- Is it hereditary?
- Do interventions work?
- How successful is AA?
- Could I be an alcoholic?
- Where can I find help?
  …and many, many more!

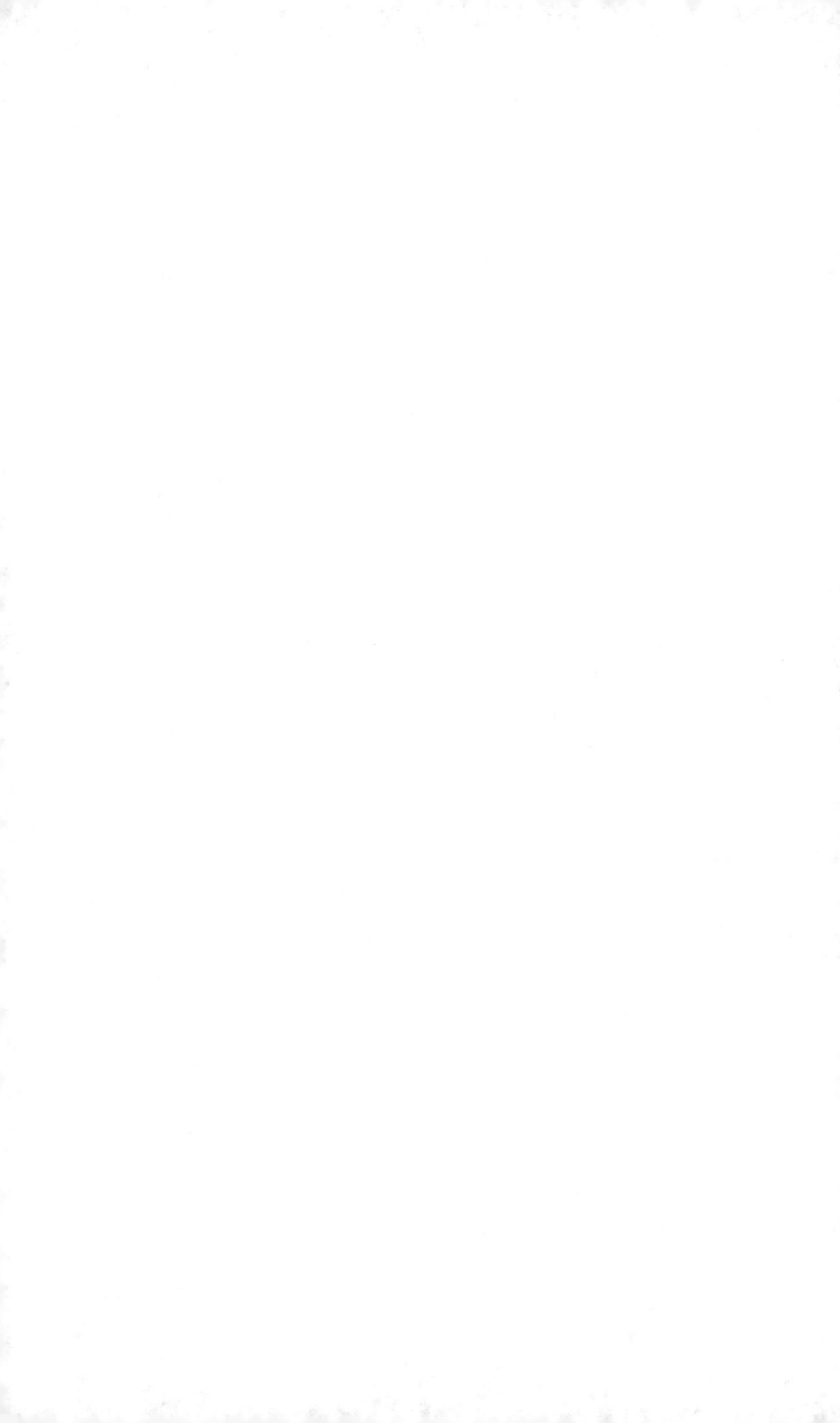

www.ingramcontent.com/pod-product-compliance
Lightning Source LLC
Chambersburg PA
CBHW060230290526
45789CB00003B/1484